RIGHT TO SEX
EDUCATION
OR A WRONG RAPE
SEX
YOGA

KORAK DAY

notionpress
.com
INDIA · SINGAPORE · MALAYSIA

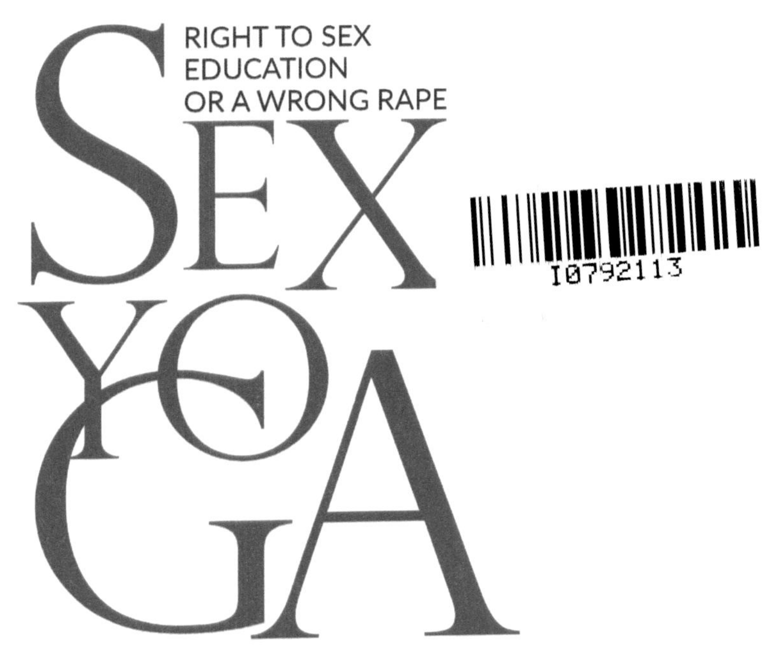

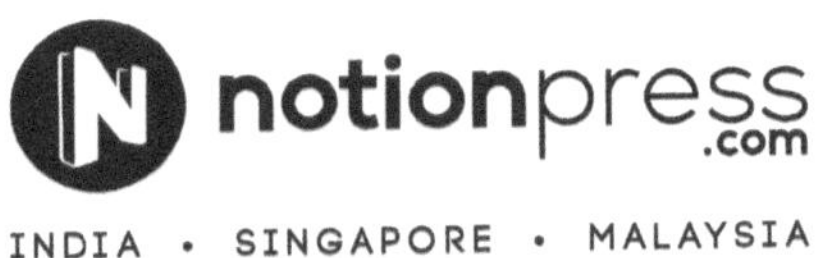

Notion Press

Old No. 38, New No. 6
McNichols Road, Chetpet
Chennai - 600 031

First Published by Notion Press 2019
Copyright © Korak Day 2019
All Rights Reserved.

ISBN 978-1-64587-542-0

Dedicated to

All those people from ancient India, for who sex was part of the divinity and they treated it like a divine offering. This to the extent of depicting the details of sex in the places, where the highest crowds came to submit themselves; the temples.

CONTENTS

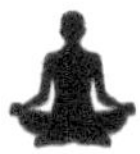

ACKNOWLEDGEMENTS

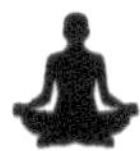

A published book is not just the contribution of the writer, I believe. So many take part in bringing it to the final version.

Dr. Dipak N Patel of USA is always the first one to thank for my Art creations, just like Theo van Gogh, the brother of one of the most celebrated artist (painter) Vincent van Gogh. Dipak's unfailing financial support allowed Korak Day to devote himself entirely to his creations of art and the works for serving humanity with selfless love.

Taking out time to create, along with all his humanitarian works that Korak does these days, would have been impossible. But there are a few people whose infinitely large selfless hearts only could make him have time and energy to create.

First two are Gopal Day and Chandragupt Day, Korak's first two Satwik Shishyays who are selflessly taking care of every problem and constraint that he faces. Gopal Day was born an Avatar whom you cannot see with Kaliyugi eyes, and the other is born Md Afzal, who is physically there. There is a third person named Koyel or Krishna Chakraborty, who was sent to me by my daughter Goddess Durga. These are the matters of soul Aatma and for the one, who has realized Aatma Yoga, can only decode this.

INTRODUCTION

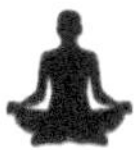

Sex is the right, which if treated wrongly can only lead to the present modern societies. Now vulgarity, rape, mistreatment of men, women and the third gender is rampant. That is done mostly by the people of the law or under the protection of the law, than the meek.

Know your body, your needs and your right to feel the ecstasy in the way that comes naturally to you. And know it perfectly, precisely and without a prejudice. This is the reason why a Satwik Aacharay has to take it upon himself to write this book.

Many would just troll you for this. The trolls would range from political to legal to the so-called intellectuals. But the Almighty and the Nature that creates all is way higher, so let the trolls take a stroll.

Know all and everything about sex. Then get to know everything about your self (maybe through my twin book, which gets published with this book called AATMA YOGA). Know they **self** within and know thy **body** firstly. And then use your **mind** to make the best use of this body towards unleashing your soul's wish. Because if you do not know your body and do not know your soul, then your mind is a rotten apple, filled with maggots. And that becomes your identity.

Wait a minute, is this the reason or the mission of the entire media and the powerful: to tame your mind by keeping you away from the sex education and soul realization? Maybe it is not and maybe its our vail on our own illiteracy. Well after these twin books of Sex Yoga and Aatma (Soul) Yoga, no one can give any excuse.

Chapter 1

WHY THIS BOOK IS A NECESSITY TODAY

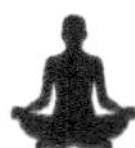

I want this book to be handy and precise. So everything would be to the point.

Media is supposed to be a medium between people and reality. But that is not how the media is at present; it's just the opposite mostly. Similarly just like we having a body is a reality and so is sexuality. The culprit is the "wrong" value systems and dictatorships of hypocrite rulers.

These rulers thought themselves to be Gods or even better, and the commoners/subjects as slaves. These idiots brought forth such stupidity about sex. Remember in India sex was depicted in the temples, where all people would come with a spiritual bow and there they would know. These rulers made such rules and laws, that made the whole world cringe in front of themselves, the humanity!

This affected so much to the entire world in a negative way. Even cultures like Bharatiya Culture or that of whatever is left as India. People here considered sex as normal in every sense of being, but they too cringed.

The rulers and the looters robbed even the Civilised Indians and now they too developed the Hipocricy Syndrome. They too would dream and do every possible sickness of sex maniac secretly, but in public, they would show off as being, better than God!

We take breadth, we eat, we drink, we are good to others or even we feel bad when someone does bad things. This is common and natural to humans. But similarly is another major thing in life, sex.

Having sex and reproduce to keep the human race away from being extinct, that too is as "normal".

Human nature as created by nature and the Almighty is based on being different.

We are beings that were in resonance with accepting the difference with peace. But evil cultures started by evil people/rulers/groups dictated even the Gods or the creator. They called some creations as normal and some as 'unacceptable'. No human being however powerful he/she is can dictate the Almighty whatever name they say.

No law/ruler/religious Hitler can dictate an individual about his spiritual choice.

This topic and talk can go on for long, but then the aim of the book gets diluted. So let us go bang in and know our body better and clearer.

Chapter 2

YOUR SIZE AND
THE RELATED SECRETS

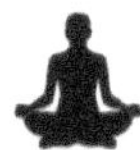

I come to this chapter with the basic essentials related to the topic of this book. I write the standards of the physical part of the 'art of sex'. Basically, this consists of the meeting between a penis and a vagina. In other situations, it could be a meeting of a penis and a penis or a vagina and a vagina.

In the act of sex then, either both or just one of them rub themselves on the other's genital organs. This in a way resulting in pre-cum. This is followed by ejaculation of semen for a man. For a woman, it would be orgiastic movements and erotic pleasure.

The sexual union, thus, demands correct length proportions of the penis and the vagina. Along with it the duration of the act and the method of the sexual union forms a major part in our learning now.

Men and women are divided into three categories each (according to the size of their penis and of the vagina).

A. Choto Man/Choto Woman.

B. Mejo Man/Mejo Woman.

C. Boro Man/Boro Woman.

Now I describe them one at a time. Know the qualities of men according to the size of their penis. This seems to be questionable, but you may do your own research for it. Just like the ancient scientists of Bharat.

FIRST FOR THE MEN:

1. The Choto Man:

    i. The Choto Man is of a cheerful nature.

    ii. He is pleasant to talk with and has a sweet tongue.

    iii. Have curly hairs.

    iv. His height is of a medium range.

    v. Has a round face.

    vi. His hands and feet are light and beautiful.

    vii. He keeps and maintains his self-respect.

    viii. Obey and give respect to his elders and authority.

    ix. His penis is around 6 inches in length.

    x. His semen emits a sweet smell.

    xi. He walks around lightly.

    xii. His sexual urges are only occasionally.

2. The Mejo Man:

    i. Like the Choto Man, he is also sweet tongued but to a certain extent only.

    ii. He has a round neck.

    iii. His voice is hoarse.

    iv. His hands and feet are red.

    v. He has a lovely gait and appearance.

    vi. His eyebrows are erect and straight.

    vii. His belly has a curve and not plain.

    viii. Both his semen and his body give away a salty smell.

    ix. He has a medium bearing and appearance.

    x. He has a taste for humor.

   xi. His penis is of the range of 9 inches.

3. The Boro Man:

     i. This is a man of a talkative nature.

    ii. His face is long.

   iii. He has long and thin ears and head.

   iv. He has thin lips.

    v. His hair is thick, crowded and curved.

   vi. He has long and muscular arms and legs.

  vii. His fingers are long and his nails are shapely.

 viii. His voice is powerful.

   ix. He walks briskly with his body.

    x. His semen emits a kind of pungent small, something like the mucus of an elephant.

   xi. He is a highly passionate man.

  xii. His penis is up to a length of 12 inches.

NOW FOR THE WOMEN:

1. The Choto Woman:

     i. In her unpredictable eyes, she has red lines in it.

    ii. Her face is round and beautiful as a lotus flower.

   iii. She has a very soft and delicate flesh.

   iv. Her breasts are full, round and hard.

    v. The color of her body is very light and white.

   vi. Her nose is as straight and smooth like the beak of a parrot.

vii. She has pearl-like white teeth.

viii. Her gracious appearance is like a swan.

ix. She speaks very sweetly like a beautiful voiced bird.

x. Her neck is also beautiful and smooth.

xi. She has great respect for elderly people and those who are more than her in knowledge.

xii. She is a very religious type of woman.

xiii. She prefers to wear white color clothes.

xiv. She likes to eat very little.

xv. She is clever in enjoyments, not voluptuous though. She knows her limits of indulgences.

xvi. She sleeps lightly and can wake up soon.

xvii. She also speaks softly and little.

xviii. The vagina of such a woman has a depth of 6 inches.

xix. The mucus discharged by her has a sweet and pleasing smell.

2. The Mejo Woman:

i. Generally, she has a slim figure, but she could also be fat.

ii. Such women are tall.

iii. She chooses to wear colorful dresses.

iv. She has a short-tempered nature.

v. Her breasts are loose, so they may hang.

vi. Her eyes could be lighter than the general and she looks at an angle or indirectly.

vii. She walks quickly.

viii. She is quite eager for the act of sex and scratching and even biting during the act.

ix. She has a taste and liking for drinking. She can be an excessive drinker too.

x. Her voice is husky and high-pitched too.

xi. She has long teeth.

xii. Her hair is straight and standing.

xiii. She enjoys sleeping.

xiv. The vagina of such a woman has a depth of 9 inches.

xv. The mucus discharged by her has a fishy smell.

3. The Boro Woman:

i. She has a kind of appearance which could be a little un-relaxed and self-conscious.

ii. Her toes are thick, fleshy and curved.

iii. Her neck is short and thick.

iv. She sports some large lips.

v. Her breasts are not proportional and thickset.

vi. Her voice is throaty and powerful.

vii. She has big-fat hips.

viii. She likes to eat salty and spicy foods a lot.

ix. She enjoys her sleep to the point of difficulty to wake her up.

x. The skin of her body has lots of hairs.

xi. She doesn't care much about others in public about her behavior.

xii. She is always ready to go through the act of sex.

xiii. She has a soft corner for earning and getting money.

xiv. The vagina of such a woman has a depth of 12 inches.

xv. The mucus discharged by her has a foul smell.

xvi. Her vagina can be stretched a lot according to the needs.

xvii. Also, her vagina is quite wide.

TYPES OF CORRESPONDENCE OF SEX ORGANS

The circumference of the penis and the vagina are according to the size and depth. The vagina can be stretched to a bigger size in all the cases.

Made For Each Other Union:

When there is a perfect correspondence between the vagina and the penis it is called 'Made For Each Other'. An example of such a 'Made For Each Other' case is between a Choto man and a Choto woman.

Love Each Other Union:

When the correspondence between the vagina and the penis is not perfect, it is called 'Love Each Other'. An example of such a case is between a Choto man and Boro woman. Here, the act of sex makes the friction caused to be so light and minimal. Then sexual satisfaction cannot be experienced as total.

When the correspondence between penis and vagina is very loose or very tight, then the pleasure of sex is the worst. The best situation is 'Made For Each Other situation. Here the correspondence between the vagina and the penis is perfect. In this case, it gives more pleasure to the female partner.

Most of the problems between a man and woman start from this kind of unequal union. This leads to other things and straying away from a man or woman from the lover/wife/husband. So it is imperative to select a partner or lover according to the above standards of men or woman.

THE SOLUTION TO PROBLEM BETWEEN UNEQUAL SEXES:

Here the correspondence between the vagina and the penis is very tight. Because of the large dimension of the penis, the woman spreads her thighs wide apart. Thus to enlarge the dimension of her vagina.

She does this so that the entry of the penis is possible.

The penis then because of the large circumference of the walls of the vagina, causes harder friction against the vaginal canal/wall. This gives a huge itching sensation to the woman.

This takes her to the Himalayas of pleasure.

Contrary to the above situation, if the dimension of the penis is shorter than the depth of the vagina, the woman doesn't get the required pleasure.

If a man or woman has enjoyed the 'Made for Each Other' situations before their marriage then they will always look out for a similar satisfying pleasure whenever they will get a chance.

This is the reason why it is important for both man and women to stay a virgin before the marriage. Or even marry their first love. Then they would know only that sexual situation with their husbands or wives. Thus they will accept that too like everything there is to in the act of sex.

TYPES OF TOUCH IN THE VAGINA:

Before going in to act of sex let us first find out about a destination of sex, the vagina. The vagina has four different kinds of touch:

1. Soft like a petal of a smooth flower. This kind of vagina doesn't need any stimulation with the help of putting the middle and the third finger into it.

2. Uneven, with a few knots on the wall. Here the insertion of the fingers for stimulation may be needed.

3. Have overhanging folds of the wall. Here also, the insertion of the fingers or stimulation may be needed.

4. Very rough just like the tongue of a cow. Here too the insertion of the fingers or stimulation may be needed.

Chapter 3

MASTER THE ART OF EMBRACING – 13 WAYS

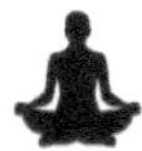

Men and women have inhabited on earth for millenniums now. They could do that only because of the acts of sex that they had been going through. All people have experienced embraces at some point in their life before embracing in the act of sex. The embraces used for the act of sex have various styles. Some of them are mentioned here below.

1. Stealing Embrace:

In this style, the two bodies only touch each other. The sensation of the other body is there but it is just for that purpose only. This style gives a major high when we are inexperienced in the act of sex. This happens by accident or intent. A man or a woman tries to pass by the side of a man or a woman. On some pretence, they would brush lightly against the body that they are attracted to. This is done without letting anybody around to suspect that it was a voluntary act.

2. Partial Embrace:

The person with some pretext or the other puts his or arm around the neck, shoulder, arms or waist of the lover. He/she chooses between holding a part of the body with a slight or strong grip. Or he/she keeps the arm for a time more than usual.

3. Initiating Embrace:

A woman is the initiator of this style of embrace. When she sees her lover in a lonely place, in the pretext of picking up something, she presses her breasts with the body of her lover. The man has the choice to either wait for another signal or he can set his hands around her body to enjoy a full embrace with her. This is done from the front or the back. Those who have still not started to talk freely with each other do the above styles of embraces.

4. Permission Embrace:

In this style of embrace, people press their body together and rub it against each other. They do it slowly and for a long duration of time. This style of embracing is done in darkness. A lonely place, a crowded place, in public transport, during a public meeting. Doing as if not realizing what they are doing, in a situation when both of them are rubbing together. Then it can lead to further stages. But in this style of embrace may be only one of them is taking part. Here the other is either quietly enjoying or testing his/her patience. Or they do not have the courage to proceed or is afraid of the situations around to respond.

5. On Your Face Embrace:

This style of embrace is a forceful kind of permission to embrace. In this style, one of the partners of the embrace stands against the wall or a pillar or a hard object for support and the other puts pressure of the body. After this, both hold onto each other making a forceful rubbing of their bodies, against their partner. Those couples that have already expressed their mutual desire for each other by some signs or a secret way perform both the above kinds. They are also both ready in their minds to perform the act of sex.

When those who meet for the act of sex, they follow the following Intimate Embraces.

6. Entwined Embrace:

A woman does this style of embrace to arouse the desire for the act of sex in a man. The effect is the same when done with the same sex. Here the woman clasps her man who is standing, from whom she desires sex. She circles her arms around him like a creeper plant around a pillar or a trunk of a tree. She looks at the face for her man lovingly and by holding the back of the neck or the head of her lower requests him for a kiss without saying anything. She also performs that in another way by clinging to the body she makes sweet and soothing sounds and talks to him with meaningful looks down at her tits. She also may look around those parts of her body that signifies a sex appeal.

7. Get Up Embrace:

This is a style of an intimate embrace. Here the woman places one of her feet on the foot of her lover then circles her other leg around the thighs of her lover. Then she presses her vagina to his penis. In another style in this embrace, she puts her arms around his waist. Then uses her other arm to pull down the shoulder of her man and amorously makes some soft and sensuous sounds. Doing thus she also lifts her body high up on the man to get his kisses on her mouth.

Both the above embraces are performed while both the partners of the act of sex are standing. Their aim is to arouse the highest passions leading to the actual act of sex. Both these embraces could be adopted in different preferences of acts of sex too.

8. Selfish Embrace:

This style of embrace is executed on the bed. Here the partners of the act of sex lie sidewise close to each other. They lie face to face and intimately and selfishly embrace each other as if they need the most for themselves from the other. The one, who is in the left side, passes the left hand under the right side of the other. And the right hand under the left arm of another and then places the left leg on the right leg of the other. In this style, the partner on the right side makes very close contact with the partner's body. Then it becomes easier to rub their private parts together. They get a euphoric JOY.

9. Intimate Embrace:

This style of embrace makes both the partners of the act of sex into one body in this style one of the partners sits on the lap of the other. Both the pairs of eyes of the lover look deeply into each other's eyes. If they are lying on the bed, the one in control grasps the other's bod. With a great force, both of them are highly in need of going through the act of sex that they want to break into each other's body and become one body. In such a situation they do not care about whether the bones of their body will break.

Both these embraces are practiced when both the partners are preparing for the act of sex. By these styles of embraces, especially the Intimate Embrace, the penis becomes erect and secretes pre-cum. Also the vagina grows wet with the pre-cum or the pre-coital fluid that prepares the vagina to accept the penis.

There are some more Extremely Pleasure Giving embraces too. They are:

10. Forceps Embrace:

The couple lies face to face in this style. One of the two partners grips either both or just one thigh of the partner. Then this one, who has gripped the thigh, exerts pressure on the other thigh. This action seems like a pair of forceps in action. The active part in this style of embrace is taken by the one with more fleshy thighs and then derives the bigger pleasure.

11. Mounted Embrace:

In this style one of the partners lies on the back, naked of course. The other partner also naked mounts on the other. Then the one who has mounted presses the legs and the waist against the body and rubs the private parts against those of the partner lying down. This is basically done to invite the other for a sexual union. Then the woman loses her hair and plays with the man's body by giving sex-bonuses to him. This movement of the embrace is for getting extreme pleasure if done properly.

12. Booby Trap Embrace:

In this style of embrace, the woman makes the best use of her breast. The woman presses her breasts against the chest of her lover. She embraces him thus throwing all her weight on her lover. In this style, the man comes in close contact with the woman's soft and fleshy breasts and experience an unending pleasure. A woman can perform this embrace by pressing her breasts on the face of the man. She can also perform the same actions by pressing her breast on the penis on the man too. This style of embrace can also be performed by either sitting posture or by lying on top of the other or side-by-side of each other.

13. Temple Embrace:

This style of embrace signifies that part of the body that is either called a forehead or a temple. Here a partner can lie upon the other whose face is looking upwards. Then both the partners look close into the eyes of each other. Then they lock their lips. Then the one on the top start to rub the temple with the temple of the one who is lying down, again and again. This particular style of embrace gives both the partners a great pleasure. This embrace could also be done while lying side by side of each other.

Embracing is such a thing that even the mention of the various embraces and the techniques arouses a desire for going through it. But the greatest pleasure comes from practicing it. As usual, practice makes a man succeed in whatever he wants.

Chapter 4

A KISS KEEPS THE EVIL AWAY – 23 WAYS

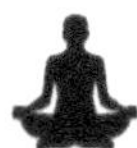

There are different parts of the world, which professes to kiss in different parts of the body and also prohibits in the other parts. But some kisses are commonplace in almost all cultures.

EROTIC KISSABLE PLACES ON OUR BODY:

i. Kissing on the temple.

ii. Kissing on the forelocks.

iii. Kissing on the cheeks.

iv. Kissing on the eyes and the eyebrows.

v. Kissing on the chest and breasts.

vi. Kissing on the lips and the interiors of the mouth.

vii. Kissing on the vulva.

viii. Kissing on the armpits.

ix. Kissing on the regions just above the private parts.

x. Kissing on the toes and fingers.

xi. Kissing on the penis and the scrotum.

xii. Kissing on and inside the navel.

xiii. Kissing on the anus and cheeks around.

xiv. Kissing on the neck and the collarbones.

xv. Kissing on the ears.

There are various other spots on the body that are kissed in different parts of the world by different people. In the general form of Kissing the lips are curved to form a shape of a bud. Then that bud shaped lips is made to touch or suck any sensuous part of the partner. The most common place of a kiss is on the lips.

Kinds of Kisses: Below we would go for the various known kinds of kisses practiced.

1. Touch Kiss:

In this style of a kiss, one of the partners persuades the other one to agree to give a kiss. Being overwhelmed with shyness the one who is a little bolder just advances the lips just to brush the partner's mouth. The other partner who is thus touched upon doesn't make any effort to press or suck the lips. None of them goes any more than this touch of lips.

2. Tremble Kiss:

In this style of kissing the ones more experienced holds the lower lip of the partner between his own lips. The other inexperienced partner who wants to respond but is shy so is unable to respond. But she cannot stop that trembling movement in her lips which is created in her excitation. Even though she does not want this but still she pretends that she wants to rescue her lips away from her partner. Then the man plays his game by trying to withdraw or at least loosen his lips. She at once fastens her own lips on his. During this phase, her lips again experience that trembling movement making the kiss pleasurable.

3. Prying Kiss:

In this kissing style, the woman takes the initiative and goes some steps further. She uses her palm to cover the eyes of her lover and also closes her eyes. Then she touches the lower lip of her lover with her lips. She slowly rubs her lips there. Then she takes the lower lip in her mouth and plays with it with her lips only or even uses her tongue. This gives her a lot of pleasure and a soothing sensation to the man.

4. Direct Kiss:

The partners of love when confronting each other they look into their eyes. They close their eyes. The man takes the lower lips of his partner between his lips. His partner does the same.

5. Angular Kiss:

Here one of the partners of love is looking to some other direction than the lover. The lover comes quietly to his partner. He turns the woman's face towards him and looks into her eyes. He then presses her lower lips with his own lips.

6. Spinning Kiss:

Here also, one of the partners of love is looking to some other direction than the lover. The lover comes to his partner. He turns the woman's face towards him with one of his hands. He uses the other hand to hold her chin. He looks for love at the whole face of his partner and comes to his destination, lips. He kisses his partner on the lips.

7. Circle Kiss:

In this style of the kiss, the man holds the lips of his partner with his thumb and the index finger. He slowly pushes both the end of the lips inside thus making the lips look like a circle. He then brushes that circle with his tongue. Later he puts his lips on the circle and sucks the circle.

8. Heavenly Kiss:

This is a very special type of kiss from the point of view of both the partners. One lover is sitting in a lower place like the ground or a couch. The lover comes from the back and looks down at his lover from the top. Either the lover sitting down looks up or he lifts the face up of his lover. The one sitting down looks up at heaven. The one standing can see the face in a reverse direction and appreciates the beauty of his lover from the point of view of heaven. He lowers his face on her and kisses on the lips in a reverse way than normal. This kind of kiss gives feelings of some heavenly pleasure that can't be felt in the other forms of kisses.

9. Loosing and Winning-Over Kiss:

This is a game of competition as who could get hold of the lips of the other's first. Both partners fall on each other in a tussle about who would be able to catch by his lips the other's lips. The man wins as the expected outcome. The woman pretends to cry, quarrel and complain that she was defeated by unfair means. She also lets the man know that he has hurt her lips badly. She turns her face from him and lies down in fraud anger. She also pretends to push her partner away from her as he comes naturally to see what has happened. Feeling guilty of hurting her the man lingers around her. He tries to soothe her by kissing her licking her and tries to turn her around to him. The woman makes use of this opportunity to ask for a second round to definitely defeat him this time. When she gets defeated this time too she shows that she is twice angry. She puts up a fake quarrel with him. The moment she finds him unawares she seizes his lips forcibly. This makes her feel victorious. She celebrates it by laughing, shouting and dancing all around. She moves her eyebrows and rolls her eyes to the man. She then taunts her partner that being a man he lost to a woman. This is a very sweet and beautiful way of getting closer in the act of sex. But this is enjoyed the most when both the partners are of a very young age.

Similarly, there are other three kinds of kisses according to the action they make:

10. Tongue Kiss:

Here both the partners' lick and such each other's tongue.

11. Teeth Kiss:

Here both the partners lick and such and bite each other's teeth.

12. French Kiss:

This is a very passionate kiss that is among the most popular and enjoyable kisses in the world. This kiss is to be enjoyed the most when given by a French who is well versant of it rather than just anyone. Many peoples claim to know it but only a few can do it effectively.

There are kisses that are according to kissing, done on various parts of the body:

13. Balanced Kiss:

This style of kiss is given on the pelvic rump, on the navel on the armpit and on the chest. These kisses are so named because they are neither too gentle nor too hurting.

14. Action Kiss:

This style of kiss is showered on the breasts and the tits, on the cheeks, on the vulva or the mouth of the vagina, on the scrotum and the penis. These kisses are so named because a lot of passion is generated while done this kind of kissing and also it is done with a lot of passion.

15. Innocent Kiss:

These kisses are very pure in disguise. They are given on the part between the breasts and the waist. Many cultures have a tradition to keep that area open while dressing up.

16. Warmth Kiss:

These kisses are done very gently and with an affectionate feel. These kisses are made on the forehead. These kisses are also made on the eyes.

Kisses are also named variously according to the situation they are given:

17. Angel Kiss:

This style of kissing takes place when one of the partners is asleep. The one who is not asleep looks lovingly at the sleeping partner. Then that partner admirably kisses the sleeping partner. This arouses a wave of passion on the one who is sleeping and in turn arouses the similar wave of surprise and passion in the other who has kissed.

18. Distracting Kiss:

This happens when one of the partners is displeased with sex. Or has become too busy to pursue the act of sex, the other one tries to distract him/her from the other works and initiate in the act of sex. The kissing in this style starts with tiny little kisses followed by getting upset of the partner. The one who wants to distract the other continues this to arouse passion by various kisses.

19. Intension Kiss:

This style of kiss is done to know about the intention of the partner. When the man has returned late and the woman is sleeping or disguising to be asleep he goes and kisses the face of the woman. This is like a signal given to the partner of the intentions. This arouses the sexual desire for the act of sex. This style of kiss is also practiced by the woman to find out whether the man wants a sexual union or not at that time.

20. Flying Kiss:

This type of kiss is generally not for getting into the act of sex. Here they use their hands or just the lips to blow kisses to their partner. This style of kiss is just when both are in a hurry.

21. Shadow Kiss:

This style of kiss is quite playful. The kiss is blown to the shadow, reflection or silhouette of the lover on the mirror water or lighted or backlighted wall or curtains. Also, the kiss could be intentionally given to a child to show to the lover. Also, the kiss could be given to the portrait of the lover. This style of kiss is done when both partners have a desire for love but are still untouched. This also tells about the state of being impatience of the man/woman for the act of sex.

22. Liberty Kiss:

Here the man or woman meets the partner suddenly in a public place. Anyone of them in the pretext of the act of sex kisses the hand of the lover. This can happen in a theater, social assembly or some cultural program where there are people who are of a certain status in the society. This style of kissing must not be done in public transport or a market place.

23. Prying Kiss:

This style is innocent and naughty at a similar instant. This is done when one of the partners is massaging the body of the other to relieve some pain or tension. Places one of the hands carefully but carelessly on the thighs of the other. Then with time one who is giving the massage puts the head on the leg and acts as if asleep. They while enacting sleep kiss the thighs to arouse passion. By this, the massaging lover conveys her mood. She does not know yet how he feels for her.

Whenever one of the lovers/partners tries to inquire about the intentions of the other then it is also the responsibility of the other partner. But if he/she does not like that at all then must not allow the other to arouse or get aroused for nothing.

Chapter 5

SCRATCH AND WIN – 12 WAYS

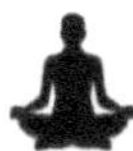

There are some particular points on the body that are much suitable for scratching. Erotic Places for Scratching:

   i. The armpit.

  ii. The breasts and the tits.

 iii. The chest and his tits.

 iv. The neck.

  v. The shoulders.

 vi. The collarbone.

 vii. The back.

viii. The cheeks of buttocks.

 ix. The pelvic regions.

  x. The thighs and especially the inner thighs.

These acts of scratching with the nail or biting with teeth are for the furthering of the act of sex. These are for highly passionate men/women. They are not to be practiced by all just because others do it.

PREFERABLE OF MEN ARE:

A man uses scratching on his partner by pressing deep his nail when they meet for the first time for sexual union. During the act of sex when the woman is intoxicated with wine, the man does it to give her a mark to remember the union when she comes out of the intoxication. When he returns to his partner/lover after a long absence. When he reconciles with the partner who was upset or angry with him.

TYPES OF SCRATCHES:

There are some basic styles of nail markings done by lovers on each other.

1. Tingling Scratch:

In this style of scratch, the nails of the man are on a medium size. He places it on the jaw or lower lip or the mount of the breast. He then presses the fingers apart on a particular part. He then presses lightly just to pinch it a little without hurting it there. This gives her an amusing tingling sensation. The hair around that part of the body stands erect. This style can be followed slowly or also quickly. This gives her an amusing tingling sensation. When we can close in the nails at the center of the lips or by the tits they naturally strike against the other making a sound. This is employed to excite a woman to a great height of pleasure.

2. Loony Scratch:

This style of scratch can be done with nails shaped round like the moon. This kind of nail is then used to prick or to press on the neck. This will also produce a great effect when done on the breasts. They sure leave some bruise marks of the shape of half moon.

3. Scratch Hole:

When two loony scratches are given near to each other while they face each other than such a full circle like hole appears. This style of scratch is generally done on the region that is hidden by the clothes generally. They are given below the navel. This style of scratch is generally done on the region that is hidden by the clothes generally. They could also be made in any part of the body too.

4. Linear Scratch:

This style of scratch also has no particularly special place. It is like scratching resembling a line. The finger makes nails line marks on the neck. They are also given on the lower part of the waist, below the navel. Lovers also use them artistically. They are also given on the lower part of the waist, below the navel.

5. Beastly Scratch:

In this style, the nail marks are made on and around the tits. They are curved in shape, running upwards, like circles.

6. Prestige Scratch:

This style of scratch is also made on the breast. Here a man uses all his fingers (nails). The scratch is made in such a way that all the marks meet at the tits putting the thumbnail just below the tip of the breast makes this mark. The other four fingernails are above the tits. Then all the fingers are drawn together to touch each other. This scratch is a mark of prestige for the woman. For a man, it requires a lot of refinement to give such a mark to his partner.

7. Pride Scratch:

Pride scratch is for that woman who regards the act of sex with pride. In this style, the five nails are placed around the tits. Then by pressing the breast thus, he draws the nails together. Many times a woman even flaunts this scratch to her friends.

8. Circular Scratch:

These scratch marks are given on the breast and waist. They are in the shape of big circles. The marks on the breasts are like that of a left shape. The scratch marks on the waist look like that of a circle.

9. Forget Me Not Scratches:

Men make these generally but also could be made by a woman too. A man gives these marks at the time of his going on a journey. He gives these scratches on the thighs and the breast of the woman in the form of meaningful lines. These are given in order for the woman to remember her husband when he is not with her and refreshes the times she has spent with him. The same also goes for a woman to a man too. For a very long separation, the lover makes four such lines. For a not so long separation it would be three lines. For short separation, it will be a line only.

According to the outline and the depth of the nail scratch, they are divided into three further categories:

1. Light & Small Scratches

2. Medium Scratches

3. Long & Deep Scratches:

GOOD QUALITY SCRATCH NAILS:

   i.   Nails with no dark or blue lines in them.

   ii. Nails with a smooth surface.

   iii. Bright nails.

   iv. Clean nails.

   v.   Nail those are neither too wide nor too short.

   vi. Nails that grow quickly.

   vii. Nails that are glossy in appearance.

   viii. Nails that are soft in nature.

People with these above techniques of scratching can invent many other kinds of scratching. The people with the above types of nails are healthy in scratching of passion. When people see these scratching marks on other people's body they grow a tendency to have that person sexually.

This is a natural phenomenon. Nail marks and dental marks are very powerful methods of arousing sexual desires. It can even arouse feelings in a man or woman who has trained themselves of celibacy

Chapter 6

BITING IS THE MOST EROTIC –
9 WAYS

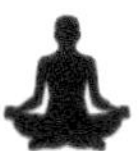

There are three places of our body where a love bite is not permissible. This is because of the danger associated. Else such sex-bites are acceptable anywhere on the body. These places to avoid are:

 i. Upper Lip.

 ii. Tongue.

 iii. Eyes.

Suitable Parts of the body where Love Bites are enjoyable are:

 i. Forehead.

 ii. Lower Lip.

 iii. The neck.

 iv. The breast.

 v. The cheeks.

 vi. The chest.

 vii. The waist.

 viii. Thighs

 ix. Pelvic rump.

 x. Armpit.

 xi. Collarbone region.

Most suitable Teeth for Erotic Markings:

  i. Even and smooth teeth.

  ii. Clean and bright teeth.

  iii. Those teeth capable of being tinted easily by some natural dying agent.

  iv. Neither too big nor too small teeth.

  v. Teeth those are closely set together.

  vi. For the sake of passion, they should have sharp ends.

Defective teeth for Erotic Markings:

  i. Teeth with no sharp ends.

  ii. Teeth that are not clean and bright.

  iii. Decayed teeth giving a foul smell.

  iv. Teeth that are not closely set.

  v. Unevenly grown teeth.

  vi. Teeth that are too large.

  vii. That that are too wide and are set apart.

KINDS OF SEX BITING & MARKINGS:

According to the dimensions of teeth, there are different kinds of sex-biting and markings:

1. Softy Sex Bites:

Here soft pressure is applied with the principal teeth. This leaves only a dim red mark. This mark only stays for some time. This indicates the initiation of sexual passion.

2. Puffed Sex Bites:

Here the biting is done with a little more force. The spot that is bitten swells up in a puff and forms a lump. This bite also stays for some time. Both the above bites are suitable in the lower lip. This bite can also be done on the cheek. Preferably the left cheek is more suitable for this biting as it gets decorated with it.

3. Beauty-Spot Sex Bite:

A very small part of the skin is taken for this kind of byte. The skin is taken between the lower front teeth and upper lip and pressed. This leaves a spot-like mark. When this bite is given on the left cheek, it makes a beauty spot mark, which looks beautiful.

4. Beauty chain Sex Bites:

When we repeat the beauty spot bites with all the lower teeth in different places it makes a series of marks. It looks very beautiful as if a small chain of beads is lying on the cheek or another part of the body. They are appropriately made on eyes, armpits and the hips. They could be made also on the mount of the breast, the pelvic rump, and the male chest. The skin in these parts is soft and can be gathered easily for passionate biting. This bites can be also done on the forehead and the thighs.

5. Clear Sex Bites:

This can be done in any part of the body. Here the skin is held between the lower lip and upper front teeth. Then it is pressed again and again repeatedly. This leaves a very clear red mark. This mark could be seen from a distance.

6. Clear chain Sex Bites:

When a lot of clear bites are made nearby each other. This byte does not cause any injury but leaves a trail of marks of red spots. They are appropriately made on eyes, armpits and the hips. They could be made also on the mount of the breast, the pelvic rump, and the male chest. The skin in these parts is soft and can be gathered easily for passionate biting.

7. Cliff Sex Bites:

These bites are made for the women's breast. A man uses his upper and lower teeth to press the top end of the breasts. This bite can also be done in another part of the cliff of her breast too. This gives round and depressed marks that are unequal in look. People of high passion practice this type of bite.

8. Chewing Sex Bite:

This byte is given mostly on the breast and the shoulder of a woman. The above-mentioned part of the body is held and chewed between the upper and lower teeth. Then another part is taken thus and chewed. Similarly, this is repeated at least five or six times in different part of the body successively. This leaves a trail of red chewed marks on the body. The very highly passionate men give this kind of sex mark. Women are also capable of giving such bytes. They do it to prove their sexual energy or their sex partner.

Some people are shy of having bruises or sex marks. In some cultures, this is a taboo.

People in some cultures are proud to flaunt their sex marks. Especially when they know that others ignore them since they are not so sexually experienced! And also that people think of them as incapable of good sex. Some people like to show off their sex marks to make people think that they are having healthy sexual relations. These people even apply artificial ways of getting these marks.

Some people even use vulgar languages and swear words during the act of sex and some people absolutely abhor them. Men and women from one culture are always attracted to those of other cultures. They know of the differences that they could experience with the partner during the act of sex.

Chapter 7

SEX BONUSES

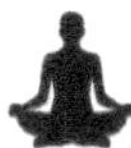

Stroking, striking and the erotic sounds are as natural as any other forms of sex-bonuses during the act of sex. There are various places on our body which when stroked, arouse us erotically:

i. The head

ii. Shoulders

iii. The area between the breasts

iv. The back

v. The tits of both man and woman

vi. The ears

vii. The buttocks

viii. The sides

ix. The neck

Parts of the Hand Best Suited for Stroking:

There are these parts of the hand which are the best suited for stroking are:

i. Palms

ii. The back of the palm

iii. The closed fist

iv. The palm and fingers extended in the full.

v. The tip of the index and middle finger the back of the fingers.

Passion Ability of the Sex-Bonuses:

There is an order of easiness and passion ability of the sex-bonuses:

★ Cooing as a stimulant is less powerful than Stroking.

★ Stroking is less powerful than biting.

★ Biting is less than scratching.

★ Scratching less than kissing as a stimulant of passion.

★ Kissing is lesser than embracing.

Order of Performances of Sex Bonuses:

But then when we see the accessibility or ease of performance they appear in reverse order as:

★ Embracing is the simplest form of sex bonus.

★ Kissing is a little more difficult than embracing.

★ Scratching is more difficult than Kissing.

★ Biting more than Scratching.

★ Stroking is more difficult than Biting, etc.

Chapter 8

MISMATCH AND AGREEMENTS IN SEX

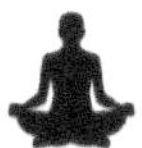

POWER OF PASSION UNIONS

1. Softly Passionate Man/Woman:

During the act of sex, this man or woman shows little interest in the process. Their moments or their progress towards the finale is also slow and weak. Their seminal fluids or orgasmic fluids are also very little. They feel embarrassed at the slightest biting or scratching did by their partner. This tendency comes due to various reasons, and one is that the person is not interested in the woman or man. Another reason for it is that they have some tension in their head. Maybe some worries they are suffering from and are unable to enjoy or take a full part in the act. Another reason is also that when a woman is more attracted to another woman than a man, she does not feel excited during the act with a man. It also goes for a man who is excited for another man only or a man more than a woman. This can also happen between two women or two men when one of them is not enjoying the act.

2. Mediocre Passionate Man/Woman:

In this category, both men and women have the intensity of passion for mediocre intensity, neither feeble nor extreme. These people are adjusting kind of people. They are more adjusting to society and relationship. These people understand the importance of a relationship where the act of sex is only a part out of many other important parts of a relation.

3. Extremely Passionate Man/Woman:

Here this man or woman has a very high intensity of passion. Their power of libido is very strong. These people can give a lot more pleasure to their partner than any one of the other categories. They know how to get what they want and they also know what to give to their partners for greatest pleasure. Many times they would not care for their partners' needs as much as they care for their pleasure. When they learn that their pleasure depends on giving pleasure, they grow up to the needs of their partners. Their seminal fluids and orgasmic secretions are also large. They have the highest tolerance for the sexual-bonuses such as scratching and biting by their partners.

One thing is very important to such people. They can use this power of extreme passion into doing something very special for their lives and for the world. People with extreme passions have always been great men and women! Especially when they choose to do something special.

According to the above intensity of passions, men and women could be put into three Identical Unions (Made For Each Other). And also for six Non-identical Unions (Love Each Other).

Made For Each Other Unions:

i.   Between Softly Passionate man and woman or man and man, or woman and woman.

ii. Between Mediocre Passionate man and woman, or man and man, or woman and woman.

iii. Between Extremely Passionate man and woman, or man and man, or woman and woman. This kind of union is considered the best total sexual pleasure.

Love Each Other Unions:

i.   Between Softly Passionate man and Mediocre Passionate woman.

ii. Between Softly Passionate man and Extremely Passionate woman.

iii. Between Mediocre Passionate man and Softly Passionate woman.

iv. Between Mediocre Passionate man and Extremely Passionate woman.

v. Between Extremely Passionate man and Softly Passionate woman.

vi. Between Extremely Passionate man and Mediocre Passionate woman.

Men and women are also divided on the basis of the time they take for the act of sex to complete.

Some take small time. Some are mediocre and some take a lot of time to complete their act of sex. Here too the situations are ideal where both partners take equal amounts of times for the process of union and thus the satisfaction. With mismatched timings, there could arise mismatched relations leading to and divorces.

At the same time lack of satisfaction can lead a man or a woman to stray. Also, at a similar breath, one can say that this lack only can lead a man or a woman to do wonders of his/her life. People in the past had been mooting over the difference of the pleasure derived by men or women. Men have a different feel of pleasure before and after they come than women.

Chapter 9

WOMEN'S SEXUAL NEEDS

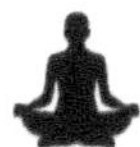

The differentiation of a woman in her feeling of pleasure is given below:

1. For a woman too, it is important to meet a man, as she too gets desperate to meet her sexual pleasures like a man.

2. It is a little different in case of a woman. Women experience a sort of itching sensation in her vagina. The hard friction can release this sensation and a penis or any other similar object, part of the body or a toy, can relieve this.

3. If this itching is not relieved then a woman can become uninterested in work, hysterical or annoyed quickly.

4. This actually leads women to enjoy masturbation like men. In the ancient cultures dominated by chauvinist men, women were denied masturbation. But they still did it secretly like the present-day women would often do, unless she is an actress.

5. A woman is known to be not only relieving her itching with the act of love but also derive extreme pleasures through the sexual-bonuses like embracing and kissing.

6. The extent of pleasure she gets is impossible for her to define and also impossible for a man to understand. This is the reason they say that a couple who kiss and embrace a lot leads a more healthy relationship on and off the acts of sex.

7. A woman starts to experience pleasure as soon as the penis is introduced even a little into her vagina. As the friction is made along the walls of the Vagina, her itching sensation starts to relieve. This feels about relief makes the woman calm down.

8. Unlike a woman's feeling of pleasure, a man feels the pleasure only at the time he comes or in other words at the ejaculation of his semen.

9. After he comes, the man tends to withdraw as the power that takes him till the ejaculation ceases instantly. This to the extent of a complete denial of any action in the act of sex. This is not the same for the woman.

10. A woman desires the movements of friction to continue even after the man's ejaculation.

11. Practically if a woman also has an ejaculation then, she may also withdraw from the man. Just like men do after he comes, without bothering whether the female partner had her full pleasure. But she does not become cold like a man.

12. A woman always loves a partner with a long duration of sustainability while she hates the short-lived man.

13. A woman likes a man with a long duration of sustainability more because he is able to relieve the woman's itch better.

14. This is a reason why many women get into a sexual relationship with another woman and a man gets into a sexual relationship with another man. Because the attainment of pleasure is more total and more with accepting the other's needs. This because they know each other's needs better than someone of different sex.

15. The above is many times untrue or is a different experience for different people. A woman generally keeps her cold before the start of the act of sex. She gradually takes momentum with the process of sexual-bonuses so by this she also experiences an ejaculation.

16. Then if she is not ejaculating then, her ovaries get activated for the start of the embryo.

17. Actually, both of them experience the gratification of sexual pleasures simultaneously.

18. It is known that the desire for pleasure in a woman is eightfold stronger than a man of a similar status of passion. This is the

reason why woman continues to need even after a man finishes his ejaculations. This is the reason men of substance prefers to go through after-plays. Even after he has had a termination of his pleasure which many times lead to a second ejaculation in men with healthy relations.

19. Both man and woman are equally active and interdependent for the proper performance of the act of sex. Unless they are of different backgrounds and preferences.

Chapter 10

SATISFYING DIFFICULT PARTNERS

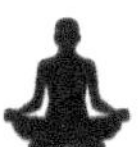

A successful act of sex:

A man's passion for the first act of sex is intense. During the second and third acts of sex on the same day, he becomes weaker and weaker with each round, on the same day. He then takes longer to be stimulated.

This case is reversed in case of a woman. During the first act, her passion is weak and takes time to be stimulated. Even with the sex-bonuses given by the man, she is not fully aroused and takes longer to achieve orgasm. On the second and better in their third rounds, she is roused and also satisfied quickly. It is quite natural for a man that he comes before the woman has discharged the fluid. This keeps her unsatisfied leading to problems.

For this problem, a man is suggested to rouse her desires first by the various sex-bonuses before he starts the actual act. In this case, both of them reach the peak of pleasure at the same time. This gives satisfaction on the act of sex and that leads to the satisfaction of a relationship.

Satisfying a difficult woman:

By the rule of nature, women are of a delicate and soft nature and are easy to be aroused. There are some exceptional cases too where the women are neither soft nor delicate.

Even handling her is simple if you are well versant of the sex-bonuses like embraces, kisses and the caressing of the orifice or the lips of the vagina.

These are the surefire inducing bonuses enough to tame any kind of women. Whether a woman or a man is of easily satisfying nature or difficult to please nature can be satisfied with the various sexual-bonuses.

Various kinds of Sexual Gratifications:

We human beings are enslaved by a particular habit of doing things. We enjoy them, and it is difficult for us to change them.

Some kind of sexual practice that we are used to doing with time gives us sexual satisfaction, again. Our imagination is a great tool that is in our reach to be used for sexual gratification. This is a gift from nature to us.

We can imagine a sexual union along with a certain action upon us or upon something else. This gives us a similar sensation. Masturbation is a kind of this type of sexual gratification.

An act of sex, done with another approachable partner making ourselves believe during the act of sex that this partner is the one whom we desire. That act which comes with the real person with whom we desire to have the sexual gratification.

A kind of sexual gratification can be achieved by watching something of an erotic nature. Sometimes when someone reads something of literature and suddenly read something of a highly erotic nature.

At a very young age when someone unknowingly touches you or someone touches you in a not necessarily sexual or erotic way. This happens when we are just new to puberty.

In all these above mentioned sexual gratification types, it depends on the personal choice of the woman or the man in what they like and what they want. Whatever they do they must see to this that they must not hurt the sentiments and one-track minds of the public.

Our personal choice is a personal choice and not a public affair. When we are satisfied and content with what we do and what we get when we have no need for bringing things up in the public.

Chapter 11

8 STYLES OF BLOWJOBS

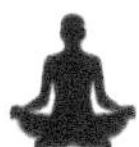

Blowjobs are of a huge fashion in modern times.

They were not so famous in the ancient time and whenever done were done in secrecy only. They are done by women and by men on a man.

Many cultures assign blowjobs to a minimal or unnatural way of having sex. The women who prefer to that are assigned as downtrodden. At the same time, many cultures assign Blowjobs as good for health.

Various Ways and Acts. There are various ways and acts of Blowjobs:

1. Lip Job:

In this method, the person giving the job takes hold of the Penis. Then rub it against the lips in slow motion.

2. Side Business:

In this style of job, the finger stretches the piss hole. The sides of the penis are pressed between the teeth and the lip slowly. This process is continued slowly.

3. Tip Top:

The woman takes the penis in her hand and puts the tip of the penis in her mouth. Then she presses the tip in such a way that the penis slips out. This process is repeated.

4. Repeat Job:

Now the penis is taken into the mouth a little more. Then it is taken in and out repeatedly. Thus, pleasure is aroused.

5. Kiss Job:

The penis is held up in the hand of his lover. Then she sucks it in such a way as the lower lip is sucked.

6. Caressing Job:

First, the lover takes the Penis in the mouth. Then the tongue caresses it. Then the wife sucks the tip of her husband's penis.

7. Concentration Job:

In this style, the woman sucks in the upper half of the penis. Then she caresses it with the tongue. Then with the skin up, she sucks it repeatedly.

8. Hide and Seek Job:

Depending on the mouth of the woman, she takes the penis in its full length inside her mouth. She then rubs it at the end of her mouth. Then she reveals it, again and again, repeats the whole process. This is done until the man ejaculates inside the mouth of the woman.

Those men who have undeveloped sexual organs also practice all these processes. This is the only way they can have a sexual union.

According to the ancient times' men used to making their servants go through blowjobs on them. Also, the old books on the sociology of all cultures also have instances where very intimate male friends resort to this practice.

Not only men, but even the ladies of the harem of the Muslim kings also resorted to the licking of each other's vulva and sucking it to derive pleasure. In many cultures, blowjobs are regarded as a health-promoting practice.

Chapter 12

ATTITUDE IS CRUCIAL EVEN IN SEX – 7 WAYS

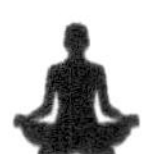

The act of sex is all about your attitude during the act. It's all about satisfying the partner and at the same time giving you full satisfaction.

Human beings and their sexual organs are of different sizes and shapes. Their level of passions are also different but at the end of these differences start the attitudes. These attitudes make us reach or leave us behind. Here is an example:

PERFECTION FOR SUFFOCATION MATCH

Perfect Attitude for a Choto-Woman and a Mejo-Man:

Let the woman lie on her back. Let her spread her thighs sufficiently wide apart to stretch her vagina to the largest.

PERFECTION FOR SPACEY MATCH

Perfect Attitude for a Boro-Woman and a Mejo or Choto-Man:

Let the woman lie on her back like before. Let her bring her thighs closely together to contract her vagina as tightly as possible.

VARIOUS ATTITUDES OF SUFFOCATION MATCH

Attitudes for a Choto-Woman for Greatest Pleasure with All Men:

1. Flowering Attitude:

The woman lying on her back raises her hips. She spreads her thighs wide apart. The woman here can also place a soft pillow under her hips. She rises up the lower part of her buttocks and opens out her legs wide apart. The vagina extends and so does the lips of the vagina.

The man places his hands under her hips to have a grip for strength. He keeps his penis between the lips of her vagina. Then he thrusts and withdraws his penis alternately slowly getting deeply inside the extended vagina.

The woman can also help the man in this by moving her hips up and down. Man must take care of the woman by inserting his penis in slow movements. Penetration must not be jerky for the sake of the man as he can injure his foreskin.

This is one of the reasons why some cultures let go of the foreskin at a small age. But it's better to have it as then as a man learns to respect a woman at least for his own sake. Penetration must be effected only after the vagina is wet with the female-fluid.

2. Gaping Attitude:

Here the woman doubles up her legs from the knees. She then draws up her thighs wide apart. Thus, both the lips of the vagina become separate forming a gap now the orifice for an outline of an opening egg.

3. Vastness Attitude:

Here the woman doubles up her legs at the knees. She draws apart her thighs in such a way that they touch the middle part of her body on the respective sides. This opens the orifice so widely that even a Choto woman can enjoy the sexual union like a Mejo woman. To master in this position a woman needs to do a lot of practice. Yoga can help widely.

VARIOUS ATTITUDES OF SPACEY MATCH

Attitudes for a Boro-Woman for Greatest Pleasure with All Men

1. Clinching Attitude:

The woman and the man lying on the bed with their legs and thighs fully spread out. Then they clinch each other with a grip. The woman opens her thighs a little to let the penis penetrate. In this position and time, the woman lying on her back can clinch the man. Now the man must lie on his left side and make the woman lie on her right side thus clinching each other.

2. Squashed Attitude:

In the above clinching attitude, the woman presses the man's thighs between her thighs tightly after receiving his penis. The penis often tends to come out in this position. The man naturally thrusts himself back into the vagina again. With the repetition of this falling out and letting in the process both the partners derive the greatest pleasure.

3. Contracting Attitude:

When the woman engaged in Clinching attitude makes a cross of her thighs with that of the man. After that, she grips the penis and holds it in her vagina. Here in this situation also the vagina is highly tightened. This the woman enjoys a lot. This result in a much greater contraction of the abdomen that gives a lot of pleasure.

4. Compression Attitude:

In this attitude, the woman is again in charge of pleasure. With her thighs, she holds the penis so tightly inside her that it is like a prisoner of war and cannot slip out at any cost. This attitude needs a lot of practice. Many sweet and delicate women generally relish this practice. Beware, men, don't get carried away by sweetness or else you would be a prisoner for life (which you will enjoy).

Chapter 13

BONUS SEXUAL UNION ATTITUDES – 13 MORE

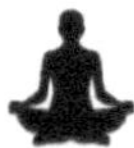

There are some more attitudes done in other parts of the earth that can help various sizes of women:

1. Up-Up Attitude:

In this style, the Boro woman lies on her back. She closes her thighs together. Then she raises her joined legs upwards. The man makes his penis touch her buttocks. Then he penetrates his penis (no not in her buttocks) but inside her vagina.

2. Shouldering Attitude:

Here the man holds the woman's thigh by his hands. He then lifts them up and makes them rest on his shoulders vertically. Then he engages in the act of sex with her. In this attitude, the thighs remain somewhat open.

3. Extra Power Attitude:

The woman lying in the Shouldering Attitude places her feet on the man's chest. The man then pulls his hands around her neck. Then they engage themselves in the act of sex.

4. Half Power Attitude:

The woman is in the Extra Power attitude. She spreads her one leg only, and the other leg is contracted against her breast. She has the sexual union in this pattern. Later both the legs can be stretched during the action, one at a time.

5. Yogic Attitude:

Here the woman rests one leg on the shoulder of her man. She spreads the other straight on the bed. Thus, she has a sexual union. During the act, both legs can take each other's place turn by turn.

6. Impressive Attitude:

A woman lying on her back raises her thighs upwards and spreads them. She crosses one leg up on the other turn by turn. Thus, she engages in the sexual union. In this attitude, the abdomen is contracted and appears tightly pressed.

7. Extra Impressive Attitude:

A woman lying on her back raises her thighs straight upwards. She crosses one leg up on the other keeping the legs up straight by making a loop. Thus, she engages in the sexual union. She may get tired after some time during the act. Then she can put her leg down by folding from the knee over the shoulder of the man who is on the act of sex with her.

8. High Thigh Attitude:

The woman folds her left leg and places her left foot on her right thigh pit (at least touching). She similarly folds the right leg and places her right foot on the left thing pit. She lies on her back. The man comes from behind the woman's knees and legs. He places his hands around her neck. Then he performs in the act of sex with her.

9. Back Pack Attitude:

Here the woman lies of her face down. The man embraces and kisses her from behind. He then introduces his penis into her vagina from behind. This attitude can be enjoyed a lot but needs a huge practice.

10. Lifting Attitude:

Here one of the partners stands up against a pillar or a wall. The other partner lifts the other bodily in his arms and starts the act of sex.

11. Riding Attitude:

The man here stands against the wall or a pillar. He holds his woman by supporting her under her buttock by encircling arising them with his palm he lifts her thus. She winds her arms around his neck. Then he encircles his hips with her legs as if she is riding on him then both have sex thus. She presses her knees or feet against the wall he is resting upon thus she swings her hips forward and backward.

12. Animal Attitude:

Here the woman bends down and stands on her feet and hands or on her knees and hands. The man entwines his hands firmly around her. Like a bull, he mounts on her. He then makes his penis enter the vagina from behind. All the sex bonuses can be performed from behind in this case too. They can imitate all the various animals and also make sounds like them. This is more for a fun attitude. People of similar sex also use a similar attitude in their own suitable ways.

13. Poly Molly Attitude:

This, when a man meets two women who love him equally or a woman, meets two men who love her equally. They perform the act of sex in turns at the same time. This can also happen when the number of women for a man or many men for a woman is more than two. One man having many wives is a common thing in many cultures even now as men also believe in their Male chauvinism. But there are many cultures that have accepted women with many husbands. Some cultures are famous for that too.

Chapter 14

SEXUAL UNION SUITABLE FOR MEN

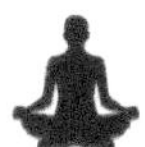

1. Universal Act of Sex:

In this case, the penis is introduced slowly into the vagina. The thrusts and the withdrawals are also done slowly. As the movements gain speed as the man approaches ejaculation. The act goes on until the man comes.

2. Merry Go Round Act of Sex:

In this, the penis is held in one hand and is introduced into the vagina. After this, the penis is churned inside the vagina in a round and round process.

3. Bite Act of Sex:

The hip of a woman is lowered. The penis is shoved into the vagina in a single rushing manner. Even with that rushing, the penis can maximally reach the upper half of the interiors of the vagina. This movement gives the feel of a bite of the penis inside the vagina.

4. Chauvinist Act of Sex:

Here the hip of the woman is raised. In a single thrust, the man thrusts his entire penis into the Vagina.

5. Violent Act of Sex:

The man introduces his penis to its full length into the vagina to its entire length. He then makes violent and forceful thrusts for a long time.

6. Crashing Act of Sex:

The man first introduces the entire length of his penis into the vagina. He then withdraws to the tip again he rams it to the full extent of his penis into the vagina. This he continues to do for some time.

7. Farmer Act of Sex:

The man introduces his penis into the vagina. He then starts to hit and dig into one sidewall of the vagina, like a farmer digging his soil.

8. Farmers Double Act of Sex:

The man introduces his penis into the vagina. He then starts to hit and dig into one sidewall of the vagina like a farmer digging his soil. He repeats that in the other wall of the vagina now. He continues to do that in both the walls.

9. Freedom Act of Sex:

The penis is first introduced to its entire length into the vagina. Then it is withdrawn a little. In that withdrawal position, the penis is moved up and down. Also, it is moved left and right. This is done over and over again along the vaginal canal. These thrusts by the penis are done at a little interval.

10. Constricted Act of Sex:

The penis is fully shoved into the vagina. When the man is about to ejaculate, the woman closes her thighs to constrict her vaginal lips so as not to let the penis slip out.

A man must not force himself on the woman and also take care of the capacity of the woman to take all those unnatural and inhuman thrusts.

Chapter 15

SEXUAL UNION SUITABLE FOR WOMEN

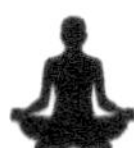

In the way a man has his way inside the vagina similarly a woman also has her way too during the Act.

1. Compression Act of Sex:

The woman receives the penis inside her vagina. Then she compresses the mouth of the vagina. Then she contracts the vaginal passage, sucks the penis inside and presses it. In this process, the penis gets imprisoned and stays for a long time inside.

2. Rotating Act of Sex:

The penis is introduced inside the woman. Now the woman makes a rotating movement making the penis to behave like an axis of rotation. This movement requires a lot of practice for the woman. The man must help in this process by raising his hips and pelvis upward to help in the movement of the woman.

3. Full Freedom Act of Sex:

A couple goes through the Rotating Act. Then the man raises his hips and pelvis up and down. He makes this movement again and again up and down and even right and left as possible.

WHEN WAYS OF WOMAN NOT ADVISABLE

The above reversed given acts where a woman was having her way is not advisable for the woman in the following stages of her life.

    i. When she is having her periods, she can suffer infertility.

   ii. She has just delivered a child, is liable to suffer leucorrhoea.

  iii. Is a Choto woman, she can get an injury due to the painful insertion.

   iv. When she is pregnant, is liable to suffer abortion.

    v. If she is very fat is useless for this purpose as she is incapable of any movement.

Chapter 16

KINDS OF MARRIAGES

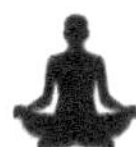

There are basically two types of marriages that are popularly known to knowledgeable people these days. These two types of marriages are more acceptable because people do know about them. There is a caveat: there are many other forms of marriage that we would read later.

1. Laudable-Prashasta Marriage:

These type of marriages are highly approved and recommended in most sane societies of the world, in today's time. This type of marriage has four sub-divisions.

- ☐ *Purest-Brahma Marriage*: Here the father of the bride would offer his daughter to a man with good moral character and is a suitable man.

- ☐ *HolyGift-Daivya Marriage*: Here the father of the bride would give away his daughter as a gift-to-God or a Dakshina. To a priest or a man of high spiritual position or knowledge.

- ☐ *Exchange-Arsha Marriage*: Here as the parents or guardians of a bride are unable to perform ceremonies of marriage. So they would do the marriage to a man in exchange for a cow, a calf and a pair of bulls, etc.

- ☐ *Responsibility-Prajapatya Marriage*: The father would give his daughter to the father of the groom, to keep as a responsibility. A Dharma, till both the bride and the groom attains a certain age to be consummated in a relationship of marriage in totality.

2. Non-Laudable-Aprashasta Marriage:

These type of marriages are highly disapproved and not-recommended in most sane societies of the world. There are many cultures and societies and religions on Earth, that promote such marriages. But this type of marraige only leads to misfortune and tragedy mostly upon the bride or groom. This type of marriage has four sub-divisions.

- ☐ *Demonic-Asura Marriages*: The father would accept money and or materials in exchange for his daughter and his son from the other party of the marriage. This type of marriage is prevalent in most parts of the world today. In some case, it is the social norm and in another case, it is the norm according to their religion.

- ☐ *Vampire-Rakshasa Marriages*: Here in this type of marriage is a case of abduction and marriage. The vampirish marriage is the one where the girl is not willing to get married to the man who was the abductor and then it is considered rape. Not only the one who rapes but also those who take part in it in any form also becomes an evil/devil for eternity. If the girl is willing, then the abduction is not Rakshasa and accepted, because a woman's will is more important than her father's.

- ☐ *Evil-Pichasha Marriage*: When a marriage takes place where the girl is married off by intoxicating her or is possessed or not in a conscious state. This is considered rape and the one who is part of this rape becomes an evil/devil for eternity. Not only the one who rapes but also those who take part in it in any form also becomes an evil/devil for eternity. Even men too are forced into such marirage often.

- ☐ *Love-Gandharva Marriage*: Here in this marriage the man and the woman do not care for their birth-givers. The family, the relatives or society or any authority and get married to each other. This kind of marriage is also a selfish and unacceptable marriage.

Chapter 17

KINDS OF SATWIK MARRIAGE

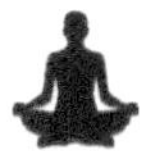

Marriage in general as we see in the previous chapter is mostly based on sex eventually to produce babies. And it happens between a man and a woman, approved or disapproved by their parents/society/relatives/laws of the land, etc.

A Satwik marriage is the third type and is totally different from the general ways of the marriages of our present times. Followings are the various aspects of Satwik marriages:

☐ Marriage here is only based on a relationship and is not based upon sex. And for the wish to producing children to help the nature or promote the family-tree.

☐ A man or a woman gets married to his work/mission/aim/art. And never gets involved in any stage of producing a baby by not even touching an opposite-sex in a sexual manner or even thinking or longing for it.

☐ Two men would get married in social marriage ways or not. But are together for a selfless cause for the benefit of humanity. Also for nature, and for spirituality, serving all three equally and truthfully.

☐ Two women would get married in social marriage ways or not. But are together for a selfless cause for the benefit of humanity. Also for nature, and for spirituality, serving all three equally and truthfully.

☐ A man and a woman would get married in social marriage ways or not. But are together for a selfless cause for the benefit of humanity. Also for nature, and for spirituality, serving all three equally and truthfully.

☐ A man who would get married or not with another man or a woman and have a child without touching the opposite sex. Done by non-normal ways and dedicate that child for a selfless cause for the benefit of humanity. Also for nature, and for spirituality, serving all three equally and truthfully.

☐ A man or a woman getting married to the divine Almighty God and gives his/her entire life for a selfless cause for the benefit of humanity. Also for nature, and for spirituality, serving all three equally and truthfully.

We have many examples of such marriages in today' times, especially in the various religious formats.

CONCLUSION

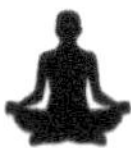

We all human beings are the Body, the Mind and also the Soul; together and not just anyone in isolation. None of the three could be denied and be of any use without the other. Most human ills take birth in us when one of the three is denied of its use/importance. In my twin book Aatma Yoga, I write about the union/connection of our Aatma, the Soul to the Divine/Almighty.

Just like getting in resonance with your soul is important, similarly getting in resonance with your body too is a major necessity. If we are not in resonance with our bodies, then we can become a monster or even turn devil/evil by performing rapes and even enjoying them.

This book is for all the men and women who are born on earth.

A healthy mind is a product of healthy self sexual knowledge. After you know the sexual side of your body, then you may choose your preference. According to your nature/desire/greed/family upbringings/society constraints. Or even spirituality/great values of service to the selfless cause, for your personal benefit. Also for nature, and the spirituality, by serving all three equally and truthfully.

Make the best choices in your life and lead a happy life. The ideal process of living a joy-filled complete life is given in detail in my book Aatma Yoga, decode the secrets within.

Chapter 18

POST PLEASURE IS JOY

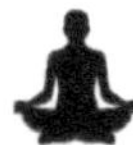

This is an optional chapter in this book. This chapter is for those who would like to take the next step from reading this book. If you want to be part of this soul-epoch and be/get a soul-dost (friend) then you are welcome to this chapter.

How you could take part in our works and missions for the benefit of humanity, starting firstly, with yourself; is the goal of this chapter.

KNOW US

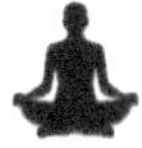

Here are our missions, our work timeline since 1996 and also some testimonials.

Satwik Aacharay Korak Day's life and works key-timeline:

Early-Life: Parmatma Prapti

Born on 1970 December 17th as Subhasish Sil in Agra, INDIA. The only son of a Para Jumping Instructor, in Indian Air Force. He studied in the Air Force School & Kendriya Vidhyalaya #1, Agra. He was the Head Boy, School-Captain. A National Champion in Inter-School level Singing and Drama. A topper in Secondary Level Exams at school-level in Hindi & English subjects. His favorite teachers were the AFS principal Ms. Sheela Jorge Russels, Ms. Kiran Basu and Mr. Moti Lal.

Later maneuvering his life, he studied until MSc. in Mathematics, at the Agra College. At the same time, he also worked as a tutor, a salesman for Eureka Forbes and Fabers. At the age of 18, he received Aatma Yoga/Parmatma-Prapti Enlightenment. That would change his course of life. The ultimate mission for a human being, to be one with the Almighty, was revealed to him.

Military Life: Satwik Renunciations

He earned the second position in the All-India Merit. That was the all-around exams for the best-educated Indian youth, the SSB. The exam was at Varanasi, for getting selected in the Indian Military as an Officer. His Training was in INS Mandovi, Goa. In Cochin, Kerala he topped in the World Leadership Foundation Course. He secured the top three awards in the first three contests only, establishing a record there.

In 1996, exactly at the age of 25 1/2, he left the Military. That was to serve Humanity & Bharat, in reality. This he craved since his Aatma Yoga Enlightenment. He arrived in Calcutta. He had renounced his most beloved foods, material-thing and everyone he knew.

Calcutta: The Christian Experience

He was Korak Day now, legally. He joined Mother Teresa's home for the dying-destitute. This was in Nirmal Hriday, Kalighat as an over-time volunteer. He started learning Indian Classical Singing, Western Piano. Also studied Films & Music theories in the USIS and NANDAN. He worked as a tutor and also joined Film Clubs. Korak lost 25 pounds in 5 months. Within a year he was selected in Satyajit Ray SRFTI. A film school for learning Film Direction & Screenplay Writing.

Soon he started going to the streets of Calcutta and Howrah Train Station. He helped the destitute there with the basics. He brought the dying-destitute, lepers and maggot-filled helpless people to hospitals. He also volunteered at Brother Xavier's school for prostitute children. At a charity school for slum-children by Calcutta De Le'rue Al'Ecole and at the local L'Arshe Home. Korak called this experience his real Ph.D. and that ended in living with the slum-dwellers.

My Karma: Awarded Film

In 2001, friends from all over the world contributed to the film created 'through' Korak Day. That was KOLKATA'R KALI alias MY KARMA (was 8.9 on IMDb). Nicholas Stroebel, France; Shaun Ho, Taiwan; John Bowman, US; David Egan, Canada. Jorge Munita, Chile; Jatin Sarkar, India, and Dipak Patel, US were the contributors. Popular Indian Film-personalities like Moonmoon Sen, Arjun Chakraborty, Sabyasachi Chakraborty acted. National Award winners Anup Mukherji for Sound. Ashoke Bose for Art and Ashim Bose for Cinematography were part of the film.

Korak Day has vowed never to accept any Award. Never for his Parmatma-Prapti Works for Humanity and Bharat. Some of the crew told him that it was not just his film only. He sent this film, to various film festivals. MY KARMA received 'Best Film' & 'Best Debut Director' Awards in 'New York Film Festival'. 'Best Screenplay' in Japanese 'Spiritual Film Festival' and a 'Grand Prix' in Poland. The film got a huge exposure, throughout the world, with 'Mother Teresa Film Festival'. Salute to the contributing friends, that such a unique film could reach humanity.

Aamar Nijer My Own Inc.: Dipak N Patel

Few months before Mother Teresa died, Korak was taken to meet her on the Saturday of the Good Friday week. There he had an out-of-body experience with her that enriched his soul. Years later on the same day of Good Friday in 2002, Korak left volunteering at Missionary of Charity. This to start his own "Mission of Love", selfless-love as 'Aamar Nijer My Own'.

This was created to care for those people who were lonely, unloved and friendless, either rich or poor. Very soon, Dr. Dipak N Patel from the USA joined as a contributing family member. Later his family too joined this Satwik Family', just like Korak's blood-parents did earlier. Without his monthly sharing, in the 'Family Kitty', all the work wouldn't have been possible. Humanity will always be indebted to his loving/caring heart!

Slums & Village Work: Islam Experience

The filth-filled and poverty-stricken Muslim slum named Butcher's Colony attracted his soul. So much that on 2002 July 2nd he started his work there. He was all alone, with no money. In a small room of the 'Torture Lane', he started teaching little children and women. In-spite of the constraints, he vowed not to accept donations. That by projecting any human being with pity. He started a 'Self- Developed

Village Program'. That in that slum for helping the women to be financially independent.

Along with four schools in Narkeldanga, had branches in three villages outside Kolkata. All turned out to be Muslim villages too. Korak was too Humane to differentiate Humans by their external ideologies. He started a 'Satwik Ashram'. This for the old, mentally-unstable destitute women and the unwanted and poor children. In a very humble way, he has made over a hundred destitute women his mother whom he calls DaDi. Meanwhile, he taught more than twelve thousand students in his 'Satwik Gurukuls'. Helped more than six hundred women & poor men mostly Muslims, to get the dignity of a job.

Satwik Art: Selfless Love

Korak created his first song 'Jiya Jae Na' during his SRFTI days, which became an instant hit. His Soul-stirring song 'Aami Manush' from his film 'My Karma' was a hit too. He continued making songs as 'Korak Gaan'. He has created 105 songs as a recording artist. Mostly Mixed & Mastered in 'Sound City' or 'BR Films' Mumbai or Film Services, Kolkata. The songs are in three languages: Hindi, English, and Bangla.

He authored and Published 'When I Visited Earth', 'Silent Symphony'. Also 'Kaamatur', 'Songs of a Satwik Soul', 'Kamokshsutra' and 'SSB Success Secrets'. Most books are available on Amazon and others online. In his Self-Dependent Villages, Korak created fashion with hand-woven Khadi-Silk. They had handcrafted embroidery & Zardozi works. He has created apparel, saris, and other products. He has also created countless 'hand-made and love-inspired' Feelings-Cards.

Renaissance: Satwik Humane

He spent six years of 'full-time' Christian experience. Then twelve years of 'full-time' Islamic experience. Post that, Korak Day decided to rejuvenate his working methods.

TESTIMONIALS

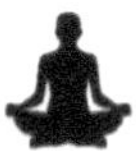

These are just a few testimonials here. You may see many more of them in the twin book called Aatma Yoga.

★ "We all made you our 'Ideal'- which we would strive to raise our standards, to behave in the way you followed every minute of every day. That's how we saw you. Korak made the concept of 'sweet sacrifice' so real, we said... Meeting you has been the most important, religious and educational experience of my life". DM, Retired Principal, Dublin.

★ "They say going to India can change a person's life", I feel this is true to a large extent. Similarly, for me, you are a large part of that- you are an important part of India. Many people say, 'Korak you are not Indian' but you embody the essence of India, too. Strong Faith and Deep beliefs. You are deep and complex... just like India's massive culture." MP, Hollywood.

★ "I always asked God to make his presence felt and through you, I felt him." Film Actress and Dancer, Kolkata

★ "I'm often not good when I speak about you. But last time I was speaking with a friend, I was speaking about your power and determination and I said: "I'm sure Korak understand something we don't know or we don't see or we don't feel." And after half a day I understand that this is the answer to the question: "Why Korak is attracting people?" You know that I have no religion, no spirituality, and no God. So I think there is a message from your soul and your heart that is transformed by your brain in determination and power. I can see that in your body, in your actions, in your words. Your brain is working well like our brain, but your brain is working in the way of your soul and heart (internal), our brain is working in the way of body and visual things (external)". NS, France

YOUR OPTIONS

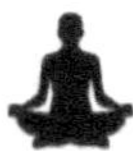

☐ Your *First Option* is to continue your life, exactly the way things were before this book. And if you have felt anything good within your soul, from this book, then our goal is fulfilled. We send you and your loved ones, good wishes.

☐ The *Second Option* is Online. You could:

   i. ☐ *Thanks*: Send us a thank you note on our email address to the 'contributors' and the 'beneficiaries' of this book. Both of them are same: the endless dying destitute around the world, unwanted children, elderly and mentally unstable fellow humans whom no one wants anymore, the lonely/friendless/unloved people living anywhere between a palace and the streets. Korak Day is just a Satwik-Medium.

   ii. ☐ *U5to5*: If you want to and feel for our soul-epoch works, then you buy five more copies of the book and gift them to five people. Then you tell them to buy five more copies each and to give them to five more people, and so on. The royalties we will get from that will be a hard-earned fruit for the beneficiaries as mentioned earlier.

   iii. ☐ *BeSoulDost*: You could choose to be a soul (friend) dost by writing to us at korakdayfilms@gmail.com or directly through the website souldost.com You would be able to get a friend who would be interested in your soul and will be a soul friend forever, online. You would be able to share, care and glare with the beauty of getting a SoulDost.

   iv. ☐ *Donate*: You could donate through our website or even directly to us in our bank for fulfilling our missions and for any of the followings: the endless dying destitute around the world, unwanted children, elderly and mentally unstable fellow humans whom no one wants anymore, the lonely/friendless/unloved people living anywhere between a palace and the streets.

v. ☐ *Volunteer*: Be a Satwik Volunteer online. You could get more info through our website souldost.com. You could be anywhere on Earth and still, you could volunteer in the soul-epoch by just taking out an hour or more in a day and serve your soul and then for others. Responsibility and commitment will be your guiding light.

☐ The *Third Option* is by meeting the Satwik Aacharay Korak Day in Kolkata, INDIA (because we do not have branches in other cities/countries now). You could:

i. ☐ *Thanks*: Come visit us and thank the 'contributors' and the 'beneficiaries' of this book. Both of them are same: the endless dying destitute around the world, unwanted children, elderly and mentally unstable fellow humans whom no one wants anymore, the lonely/friendless/ unloved people living anywhere between a palace and the streets. Korak Day is just a Satwik-Medium. Spend a few hours with our Humane-Family.

ii. ☐ *Volunteer*: Be a Satwik Volunteer in any of our present works according to your talent and wishes. You could get more info through our website souldost.com. Responsibility and commitment will be your guiding light. You could choose from 2 Days to 2 Years of various volunteering options, with or without stay/food and similarly with/without paying options. Conditions applied.

iii. ☐ *Donate*: You could donate directly to our designated Satwik Manager or even directly to us in our bank for fulfilling our missions and for any of the followings: the endless dying destitute around the world, unwanted children, elderly and mentally unstable fellow humans whom no one wants anymore, the lonely/friendless/unloved people living anywhere between a palace and the streets.

iv. ☐ *BuildAlong*: We have projects running for building infrastructure and Satwik-Homes for our Humane-Family towards fulfilling our missions. Here you may Contribute/ Donate/Buy according to the latest schemes available. You will get to know more details below and on the website.

v. ☐ *HomeStay*: This is an interesting option where you can stay in your Soul-Home in our branches and we would be happy to be hospitable to you and your family. You could enjoy Satwik meals and an environment which is other-worldly. Here too you may Contribute/Donate/Buy according to the latest schemes available. You will get to know more details below and on the website.

vi. ☐ *ARTpatron*: This option is for those who are Art lovers and can appreciate and differentiate a piece of art from a product. We create films, music, books, etc and you could Contribute/ Donate/Buy according to the latest schemes available. You will get to know more details below and on the website.

Our Upcoming Projects

#1 **SOULDOST HOMESTAY**: Be a part of Souldost-Homes [A HomeStay for you away from your own home, a Vanaprastha-Home for the affluent elderly, a Second Home as a permanent/temporary home for the rich-handicapped, a Conference Hall, a Picnic Spot, a Satwik Kitchen and a Satwik Family-Home for 50 elderly female Destitute]. We are constructing this project already, but due to lack of sufficient funds, it is taking a very long time. You could cheer this project up, with your generous contributions with/without getting benefits as you would find below and also on our website.

Total Budget is $ 2 Million or Indian Rupee 12.5 Crore. You could either 'Donate Freely' or 'Get a Return Gift.' More details will be on our website. Meanwhile, if you want to donate freely, we are giving our bank details below.

The *'Get a Return Gift'* option for this Project is:

#1 You Donate Rs. 60/$1 – Download a Certificate

#2 You Donate Rs. 1000/$ 15 – Download a Certificate + 05% Discount on Your HomeStays Rent + 05% on Food (02 days/year) Conditions Applied.

#3 You Donate Rs. 50,000/$750 – Certificate Sent to Your Mailing Address + 10% Discount on Your HomeStays Rent + 05% on Food (10 days/year) Conditions Applied.

#4 You Donate Rs. 2 Lakh/$2,900 – Certificate Sent to Your Mailing Address + 25% Discount on Your HomeStays Rent + 10% on Food (10 days/year) Conditions Applied.

#5 You Donate Rs. 5 Lakh/$7,250 – Certificate Sent to Your Mailing Address + 50% Discount on Your HomeStays Rent + 15% on Food (10 days/year) Conditions Applied.

#6 You Donate Rs. 20 Lakh/$28,900 – Certificate Sent to Your Mailing Address + 75% Discount on Your HomeStays Rent + 20% on Food (10 days/year) Conditions Applied.

#7 You Donate Rs. 50 Lakh/$72,200 – Certificate Sent to Your Mailing Address + 95% Discount on Your HomeStays Rent + 45% on Food (05 days/year) Conditions Applied.

#8 You Donate Rs. 75 Lakh/$108,300 – Certificate Sent to Your Mailing Address + 95% Discount on Your HomeStays Rent + 45% on Food (08 days/year) Conditions Applied.

#9 You Donate Rs. 1 Crore/$144,400 – Certificate Sent to Your Mailing Address + 95% Discount on Your HomeStays Rent + 45% on Food (12 days/year) Conditions Applied.

#10 You Donate Rs. 2 Crore/$288,800 – Certificate Sent to Your Mailing Address + 95% Discount on Your HomeStays Rent + 45% on Food (26 days/year) Conditions Applied.

#11 You Donate Rs. 7 Crore/$1,000,000 – Certificate Sent to Your Mailing Address + 95% Discount on Your HomeStays Rent + 45% on Food (80 days/year) Conditions Applied.

#2 HARI DHAAM TEMPLE: A Satwik & Secular Vishnu Temple with all his Avatars [a Satwik Hari Temple, a Gau–Shala for Indian–breed cows, a Ceremony Hall for festivals to enrich our souls, a Hari's Garden and a Family-Home for 50 elderly male Destitute & a Hari's Kitchen for delicious soul-satisfying foods]. We are constructing this project already, but due to lack of sufficient funds, it is taking a very long time. You could cheer this project up, with your generous contributions with/without getting benefits as you would find below and also on our website.

Total Budget is $ 850,000 or Indian Rupee 5.5 Crore. You could either 'Donate Freely' or 'Get a Return Gift.' More details will be on our website. Meanwhile, if you want to donate freely, we are giving our bank details below.

The '*Get a Return Gift*' option for this Project is:

#1 You Donate Rs. 101/$2 – Download a Certificate

#2 You Donate Rs. 1001/$ 15 – Certificate Sent to Your Mailing Address.

#3 You Donate Rs. 50,001/$750 – Certificate Sent to Your Mailing Address + Your Chosen Name+City/Town will be written on the back side brick of the Temple so that anyone going to that side can see. Conditions Applied.

#4 You Donate Rs. 2 Lakh/$2,900 – Certificate Sent to Your Mailing Address + Your Chosen Name+ Full Address will be written on the side brick of the Temple so that anyone going to that side can see. Conditions Applied.

#5 You Donate Rs. 5 Lakh/$7,250 – Certificate Sent to Your Mailing Address + Your Chosen Name+City/Town will be written on a side pillar of the Temple so that anyone going to that side can see. Conditions Applied.

#6 You Donate Rs. 20 Lakh/$28,900 – Certificate Sent to Your Mailing Address + Your Chosen Name+ Full Address will be written on a side pillar of the Temple so that anyone going to that side can see. Conditions Applied.

#7 You Donate Rs. 50 Lakh/$72,200 – Certificate Sent to Your Mailing Address + Your Chosen Name+City/Town will be written on the front pillar of the Temple so that everyone can see. Conditions Applied.

#8 You Donate Rs. 75 Lakh/$108,300 – Certificate Sent to Your Mailing Address + Your Chosen Name+ Full Address will be written on the front pillar of the Temple so that everyone who enters can see. Conditions Applied.

#9 You Donate Rs. 1 Crore/$144,400 – Certificate Sent to Your Mailing Address + Your Chosen Name+City/Town will be prominently placed in the entrance of the Temple so that everyone who enters can see. Conditions Applied.

#10 You Donate Rs. 2 Crore/$288,800 – Certificate Sent to Your Mailing Address + Your Chosen Name+ Full Address will be prominently placed in the entrance of the Temple so that everyone who enters can see. Conditions Applied.

#3 **ART PATRON**: Entertainment and Beyond inspired Films, Songs, Books created for Giving the elderly destitute and unwanted children a caring-family [3 feature Films, 15 Short Films, and 75 Music Videos]. We are creating arts in this project already, but due to lack of sufficient funds, it is taking a very long time. You could cheer this project up, with your generous contributions with/ without getting benefits as you would find below and also on our website.

Total Budget is $ 4 Million or Indian Rupee 26 Crore. You could either 'Donate Freely' or 'Get a Return Gift.' More details will be on our website. Meanwhile, if you want to donate freely, we are giving our bank details below.

The *'Get a Return Gift'* option for this Project is:

#1 You Donate Rs. 60/$1 – Download a Certificate

#2 You Donate Rs. 1000/$ 15 – Certificate Sent to Your Mailing Address + MORE (Many more benefits will come to you as this project becomes fulfilled, which you would be notified. Here you have to share on good faith, and you will receive well). Conditions Applied.

#3 You Donate Rs. 50,000/$750 – Certificate Sent to Your Mailing Address + Co-Producer Credit for one of our Feature Film + 0.03% Share of Profits + MORE (Many more benefits will come to you as this project becomes fulfilled, which you would be notified. Here you have to share on good faith, and you will receive well. The returns will be given until 20 years from the date of the film's release). Conditions Applied.

#4 You Donate Rs. 2 Lakh/$2,900 – Certificate Sent to Your Mailing Address + Co-Producer Credit for one of our Feature Film + 0.12% Share of Profits + MORE (Many more benefits will come to you as this project becomes fulfilled, which you would be notified. Here you have to share on good faith, and you will receive well. The returns will be given until 20 years from the date of the film's release). Conditions Applied.

#5 You Donate Rs. 5 Lakh/$7,250 – Certificate Sent to Your Mailing Address + Co-Producer Credit for one of our Feature Film + 0.30% Share of Profits + MORE (Many more benefits will come to you as this project becomes fulfilled, which you would be notified. Here you have to share on good faith, and you will receive well. The returns will be given until 20 years from the date of the film's release). Conditions Applied.

#6 You Donate Rs. 20 Lakh/$28,900 – Certificate Sent to Your Mailing Address + Co-Producer Credit for one of our Feature Film + 1.05% Share of Profits + MORE (Many more benefits will come to you as this project becomes fulfilled, which you would be notified. Here you have to share on good faith, and you will receive well. The returns will be given until 20 years from the date of the film's release). Conditions Applied.

#7 You Donate Rs. 50 Lakh/$72,200 – Certificate Sent to Your Mailing Address + Co-Producer Credit for one of our Feature Film + 2.25% Share of Profits + MORE (Many more benefits will come to you as this project becomes fulfilled, which you would be notified. Here you have to share on good faith, and you will receive well.

The returns will be given until 20 years from the date of the film's release). Conditions Applied.

#8 You Donate Rs. 75 Lakh/$108,300 – Certificate Sent to Your Mailing Address + Co-Producer Credit for one of our Feature Film + 3.25% Share of Profits + MORE (Many more benefits will come to you as this project becomes fulfilled, which you would be notified. Here you have to share on good faith, and you will receive well. The returns will be given until 20 years from the date of the film's release). Conditions Applied.

#9 You Donate Rs. 1 Crore/$144,400 – Certificate Sent to Your Mailing Address + Co-Producer Credit for one of our Feature Film + 4.5% Share of Profits + MORE (Many more benefits will come to you as this project becomes fulfilled, which you would be notified. Here you have to share on good faith, and you will receive well. The returns will be given until 20 years from the date of the film's release). Conditions Applied.

#10 You Donate Rs. 2 Crore/$288,800 – Certificate Sent to Your Mailing Address + Co-Producer Credit for one of our Feature Film + 9% Share of Profits + MORE (Many more benefits will come to you as this project becomes fulfilled, which you would be notified. Here you have to share on good faith, and you will receive well. The returns will be given until 20 years from the date of the film's release). Conditions Applied.

#11 You Donate Rs. 7 Crore/$1,000,000 – Certificate Sent to Your Mailing Address + Co-Producer Credit for one of our Feature Film + 17% Share of Profits + MORE (Many more benefits will come to you as this project becomes fulfilled, which you would be notified. Here you have to share on good faith, and you will receive well. The returns will be given until 20 years from the date of the film's release). Conditions Applied.

#12 You Donate Rs. 18 Crore/$2,500,000 – Certificate Sent to Your Mailing Address + Co-Producer Credit for one of our Feature Film + 40% Share of Profits + MORE (Many more benefits will come to you as this project becomes fulfilled, which you would be notified. Here you have to share on good faith, and you will receive well. The returns will be given until 20 years from the date of the film's release). Conditions Applied.

OUR CONTACT AND BANK DETAILS

Our contact address is:

Korak Day
c/o SATWIK HUMANE
3/3 Gauri Shankar Ghosal Lane,
Sastitala,
PO Narkeldanga
Kolkata 700011
INDIA
korakdayfilms@gmail.com

Bank Details for donations (we still do not have tax deduction benefits and the foreign currency accepting legal documents here yet, so you could use other options):

1. Name of Account: SATWIK HUMANE (for donors in India only)
    Name of Bank: Bandhan Bank
    Account Number: 10180006352326
    IFS Code: BDBL0001022
    Swift Code: BNDNINCC

2. Name of Account: KORAK DAY (for all currencies)
    Name of Bank: HDFC BANK
    Account Number: 50100167432320
    IFS Code: HDFC0001224
    Swift Code: HDFCINBBCAL

When you are donating money directly to Korak Day's account, it makes the transactions smooth and, when you mention that you are giving the money as a LOAN. Whatever way you Donate/Give/Contribute, all the funds will go for our missions of serving humanity, only:

If you are contributing to our ART Project as an ARTpatron, then you can give us directly to our Company's Bank Account as below.

3. Name of Account: SATWIK HUMANE
    Name of Bank: HDFC BANK
    Account Number: 50200032726640
    IFS Code: HDFC0001224
    Swift Code: HDFCINBBCAL

Also, you may send us a Cheque to "Korak Day" or Western Union Money Transfer in the same name.

Other Books of KORAK DAY

SSB SUCCESS SECRETS
(Amazon #1 Bestseller)

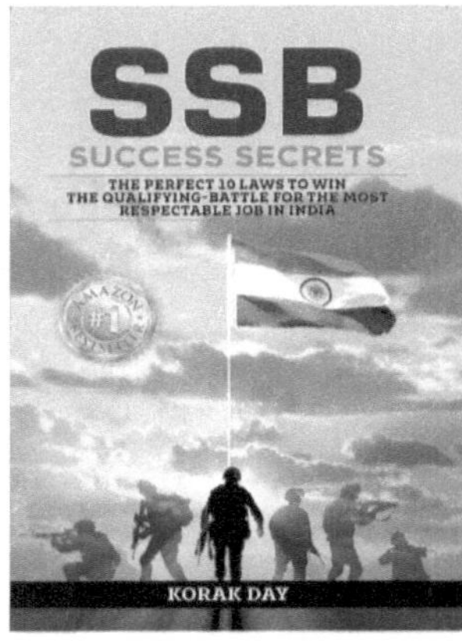

KAAMATUR

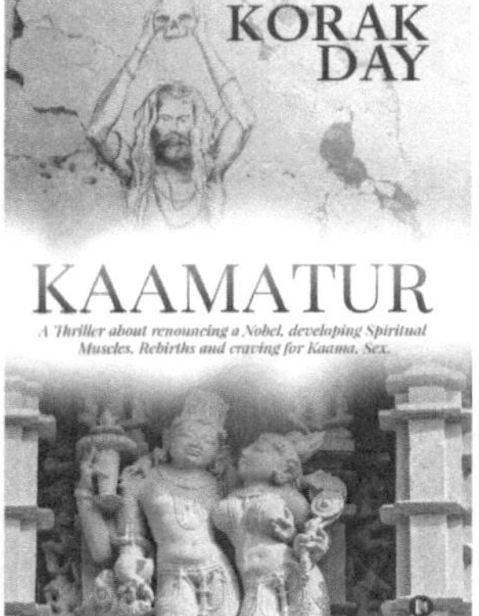

WHEN I VISITED EARTH

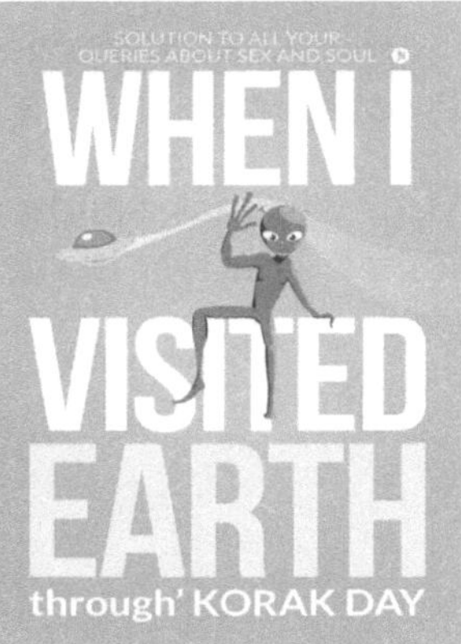

SONGS OF A SATWIK SOUL
(A Book of Poetries)

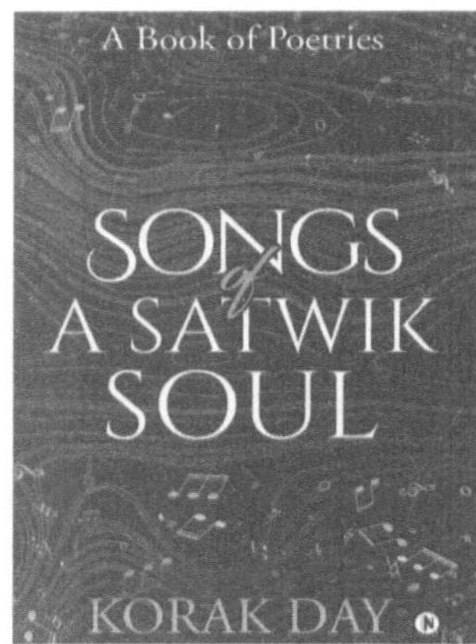

KAMOKSHSUTRA

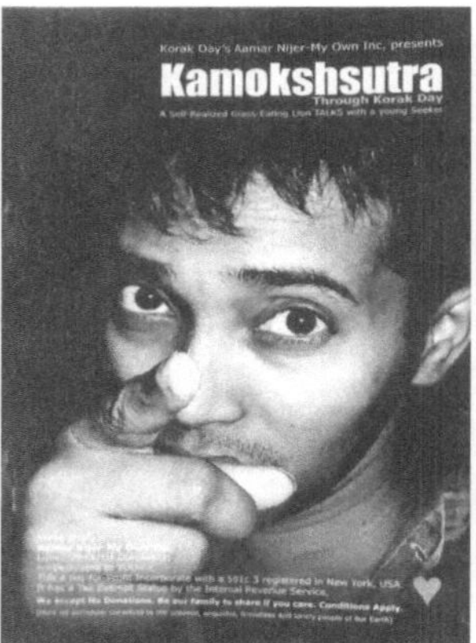

THE SILENT SYMPHONY

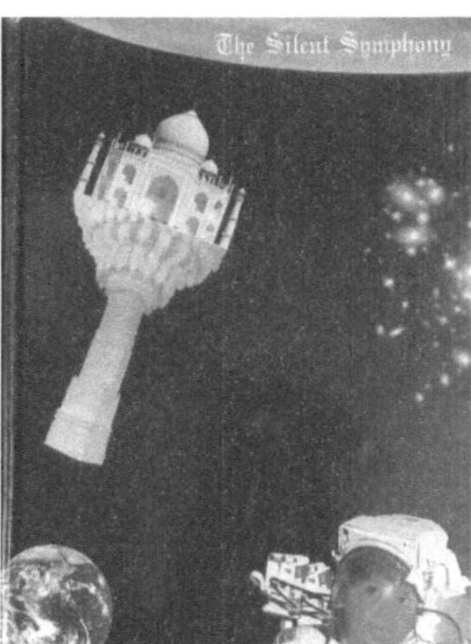

AATMA YOGA

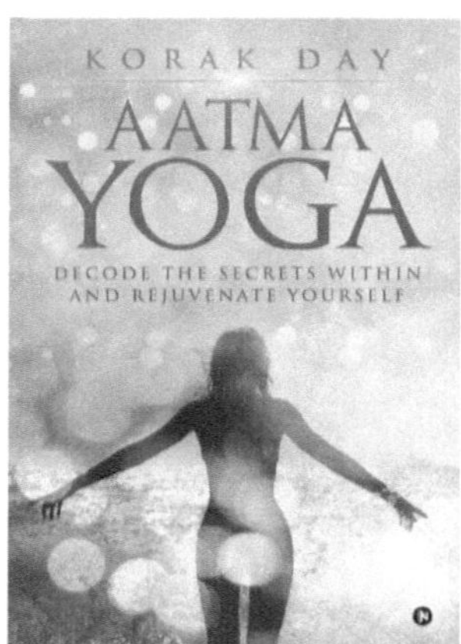

www.ingramcontent.com/pod-product-compliance
Lightning Source LLC
Chambersburg PA
CBHW031149250726
48655CB00002B/902